My fitness

JOURNAL

on my way to

NEW HABITS, NEW ME

THIS JOURNAL BELONGS TO:

_____

Name

MY JOURNEY STARTS ON:

_____

Date

LETTER FROM THE FOUNDERS

Welcome!

We are so happy to have you here and are super excited to see you start this journey to a healthier you!

Just a little background about the faces behind this fitness journal, my husband and I are the co-founders of RIMSports!

We created this brand of sporting goods and accessories because of our shared love for fitness and for each other (yes, cheesy I know).

It all started four years ago when we decided to workout at our local gym after struggling with failed diets and fluctuating weight gain. We both desperately needed to improve our health because of a history of illness in our families and the damaging habits we were creating for ourselves and future generations.

Because it had been a while since we visited a gym, I wanted to match my workout gloves with my outfit (because doesn't everyone)! Failing to find any vibrant colors other than black, Colin found a way to make a pair of pink gloves and surprised me with the first ever RIMSports Weightlifting Gloves.

Over the years, we as a small-family business have made the values of hard work, vision, and focus our guiding principles.

We spend every waking moment creating higher quality and more durable products for our customers that we would be confident to use and proud to wear.

After talking with industry experts, fitness trainers, body-builders, and our loyal customers, we have devised an all-encompassing way to track your fitness goals alongside your weight loss progress. There is no comparable fitness guide on the market that lets you record your max reps next to your meals!

You see, we are just like you. We struggled with our inability to stick to our daily workout and eating schedules. This is why we created this journal - to stay accountable. We hope you find value in not only our story but this fitness journal and meal planner, as you take this bold step towards breaking unhealthy habits and living your best life!

Ever humbly yours,

Colin & Angie

WHAT ARE EXPERTS SAYING ABOUT THIS JOURNAL?

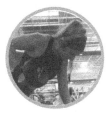

Kara Sakievich | Spring, TX

Having a single place to track all my information is so helpful. When I can see the data, I can remove my own drama so that I can really measure how I'm following through and creating sustainable changes. RIMSports has outcome. There's something powerful about writing it down daily and I'm so glad to have this useful tool to not only help me create self awareness but to encourage me to see victories beyond the scale.

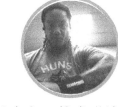

Jordan Stevens | Sterling Heights, MI

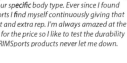

This journal is a super effective way to get the maximum documentation of your fitness journey. It will help you track and understand what's working for your specific body type. Ever since I found RIMSports I find myself continuously giving that extra set and extra rep. I'm always amazed at the quality for the price so I like to test the durability and RIMSports products never let me down.

Lindsey Yazzie | Long Lake, MN

I admire how RIMSports listens to ALL feedback and implements those changes into their products; you can tell how much their customers mean to them! I'm a visual person, so I am excited to use this journal! It will help me stay accountable because it allows me to have all my information in one place.

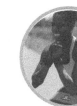

Shante Lesoken | Suffolk, VA

In my fitness journey I always tell myself success is the sum of small efforts repeated day in and day out. This fitness journal helps me keep track of all my efforts in one place. RimSports products are also a reminder that effort put in little details that other products lack makes a difference. They help me become stronger everyday stylishly and, most importantly safely. I am proud to be apart of the RIMSports tribe.

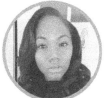

Jay Barton-Dickens | Baltimore, MD

Keeping track of my caloric intake was extremely helpful when I was trying to lose weight. I've loss over 30 pounds just by following a clean diet plan. Having a daily journal is great for those that's on their journey to a healthier lifestyle. Having one journal to log workouts, meals and water intake is very convenient. I wish I had a journal from RIMSports when I rst started my tness journal. I have several note pads with my Youtube Channel ideas, meal prep plans, recipes, body measurements and motivational quotes. With a journal from RIMSports I'm able to condense everything into one book. Remember the only impossible journey is the one you never begin.

CROSS A BIG "X"

OVER EACH DAY YOU COMPLETE YOUR DAILY GOALS

1	2	3	4	5	6	7	8	9	10
11	12	13	14	15	16	17	18	19	20
21	22	23	24	25	26	27	28	29	30
31	32	33	34	35	36	37	38	39	40
41	42	43	44	45	46	47	48	49	50
51	52	53	54	55	56	57	58	59	60
61	62	63	64	65	66	67	68	69	70
71	72	73	74	75	76	77	78	79	80
81	82	83	84	85	86	87	88	89	90

D A Y S

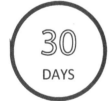

30 DAYS

Break
Unhealthy
Habits!

60 DAYS

Celebrate
Your
Progress!

90 DAYS

Enjoy
Your
Success!

BODY MEASUREMENTS

MEASUREMENT GUIDE

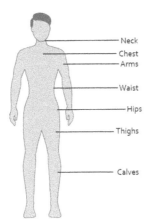

- Neck
- Chest
- Arms
- Waist
- Hips
- Thighs
- Calves

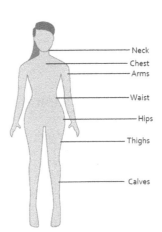

- Neck
- Chest
- Arms
- Waist
- Hips
- Thighs
- Calves

PROGRESS TRACKER

	Today	Week 1	Week 2	Week 3	Week 4	Week 5	Week 6	Week 7	Week 8	Week 9	Week 10	Week 11	Week 12	Week 13
Neck														
Chest														
Arms														
Waist														
Hips														
Thighs														
Calves														
Weight														
Body Fat														
Other														

TIPS
Use a flexible measuring tape, such as plastic or cloth.
When taking measurements, stand tall with your muscles relaxed and feet together.

TIPS
Apply constant pressure to the tape (so it doesn't sag) without pinching the skin.
Measure under the same conditions each time, such as wearing the same clothes (or none at all).

TIPS
Measure yourself in front of a mirror to make sure the tape is positioned correctly. If possible, have someone else do the measuring for you.

How I feel today

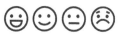

"The secret of getting ahead is getting started."
- Agatha Christie

DAY **1**

Date_____

MY COMMITMENTS

_____

_____

_____

FOOD	BREAKFAST	LUNCH	DINNER	SNACKS
	_____	_____	_____	_____
	_____	_____	_____	_____
	_____	_____	_____	_____
	_____	_____	_____	_____
	_____	_____	_____	_____
	CALORIES :	CALORIES :	CALORIES :	CALORIES :

WEIGHTS & REPS		FATS	CARBS	PROTEINS

FITNESS	WATER IN TAKE	CALORIES	SLEEP TIME	WAKE UP TIME	WEIGHT
	🥛🥛🥛🥛🥛🥛🥛				
MIN / HRS					

MY ACHIEVEMENTS
☐ _____
☐ _____
☐ _____

How I feel today

"The human body is the only machine for which there are no spare parts."
- Hermann M. Biggs

DAY **2**

Date_____

MY COMMITMENTS

_____

_____

_____

	BREAKFAST	LUNCH	DINNER	SNACKS
FOOD	_____	_____	_____	_____
	_____	_____	_____	_____
	_____	_____	_____	_____
	_____	_____	_____	_____
	_____	_____	_____	_____
	CALORIES :	CALORIES :	CALORIES :	CALORIES :

WEIGHTS & REPS		FATS	CARBS	PROTEINS

FITNESS	WATER IN TAKE	CALORIES	SLEEP TIME	WAKE UP TIME	WEIGHT
	🥛🥛🥛🥛🥛🥛🥛				
MIN / HRS					

MY ACHIEVEMENTS
☐ _____
☐ _____
☐ _____

How I feel today

😀 🙂 😐 🙁

DAY **3**

Date_____

MY COMMITMENTS

_____
_____
_____

	BREAKFAST	LUNCH	DINNER	SNACKS
FOOD				
	CALORIES :	CALORIES :	CALORIES :	CALORIES :

WEIGHTS & REPS		FATS	CARBS	PROTEINS

FITNESS	WATER IN TAKE	CALORIES	SLEEP TIME	WAKE UP TIME	WEIGHT
MIN / HRS	🥛🥛🥛🥛🥛🥛🥛🥛				

MY ACHIEVEMENTS

☐ _____
☐ _____
☐ _____

How I feel today

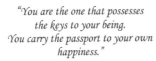

"You are the one that possesses the keys to your being. You carry the passport to your own happiness."
- Dianevon Furstenberg

DAY **4**

Date_____

MY COMMITMENTS

_____

_____

_____

	BREAKFAST	LUNCH	DINNER	SNACKS
FOOD				
	CALORIES :	CALORIES :	CALORIES :	CALORIES :

WEIGHTS & REPS	FATS	CARBS	PROTEINS

FITNESS	WATER IN TAKE	CALORIES	SLEEP TIME	WAKE UP TIME	WEIGHT
MIN / HRS					

MY ACHIEVEMENTS
☐ _____
☐ _____
☐ _____

How I feel today

"Make the most of yourself by fanning the tiny, inner sparks of possibility into flames of achievement."
- Golda Meir

DAY **5**

Date_____

MY COMMITMENTS

_____
_____
_____

	BREAKFAST	LUNCH	DINNER	SNACKS
FOOD	_____ _____ _____ _____ _____	_____ _____ _____ _____ _____	_____ _____ _____ _____ _____	_____ _____ _____ _____ _____
	CALORIES :	CALORIES :	CALORIES :	CALORIES :

WEIGHTS & REPS		FATS	CARBS	PROTEINS

FITNESS	WATER IN TAKE	CALORIES	SLEEP TIME	WAKE UP TIME	WEIGHT
MIN / HRS					

MY ACHIEVEMENTS
☐ _____
☐ _____
☐ _____

How I feel today

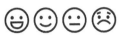

"I didn't get there by wishing for it or hoping for it, but by working for it."
- Estee Laude

DAY **6**

Date_____

MY COMMITMENTS

_____
_____
_____
_____

FOOD	BREAKFAST	LUNCH	DINNER	SNACKS
	_____	_____	_____	_____
	_____	_____	_____	_____
	_____	_____	_____	_____
	_____	_____	_____	_____
	_____	_____	_____	_____
	CALORIES :	CALORIES :	CALORIES :	CALORIES :

WEIGHTS & REPS			FATS	CARBS	PROTEINS

FITNESS	WATER IN TAKE	CALORIES	SLEEP TIME	WAKE UP TIME	WEIGHT
MIN / HRS	🥛🥛🥛🥛🥛🥛🥛				

MY ACHIEVEMENTS
☐ _____
☐ _____
☐ _____

How I feel today

😃 🙂 😐 😣

"The most difficult thing is the decision to act, the rest is merely tenacity."
- Amelia Earhart

DAY **7**

Date_____

MY COMMITMENTS

_____
_____
_____
_____

FOOD	BREAKFAST	LUNCH	DINNER	SNACKS
	_____	_____	_____	_____
	_____	_____	_____	_____
	_____	_____	_____	_____
	_____	_____	_____	_____
	_____	_____	_____	_____
	CALORIES :	CALORIES :	CALORIES :	CALORIES :

WEIGHTS & REPS		FATS	CARBS	PROTEINS

FITNESS	WATER IN TAKE	CALORIES	SLEEP TIME	WAKE UP TIME	WEIGHT
	🥛🥛🥛🥛🥛🥛🥛				
MIN / HRS					

MY ACHIEVEMENTS
☐ _____
☐ _____
☐ _____

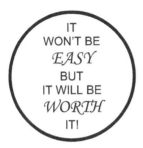

IT
WON'T BE
EASY
BUT
IT WILL BE
WORTH
IT!

WEEKLY CHECK IN

CHECK IN

	M	T	W	T	F	S	S
Drink 8 glasses water	☐	☐	☐	☐	☐	☐	☐
Take my vitamins / supplements	☐	☐	☐	☐	☐	☐	☐
Do my cardio workout	☐	☐	☐	☐	☐	☐	☐
Completed my strength training	☐	☐	☐	☐	☐	☐	☐
Recorded in my food journal	☐	☐	☐	☐	☐	☐	☐
Measured my weight	☐	☐	☐	☐	☐	☐	☐
	☐	☐	☐	☐	☐	☐	☐

DID YOU ACCOMPLISH LAST WEEK'S GOALS? IF NOT, WHY?

_____

_____

_____

_____

NEXT WEEK'S GOALS

☐ _____

☐ _____

☐ _____

☐ _____

How I feel today

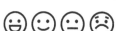

"I have stood on a mountain of no's for one yes."
- B. Smith

DAY **8**

Date_____

MY COMMITMENTS

_____

_____

_____

FOOD	BREAKFAST	LUNCH	DINNER	SNACKS
	CALORIES :	CALORIES :	CALORIES :	CALORIES :

WEIGHTS & REPS	FATS	CARBS	PROTEINS

FITNESS	WATER IN TAKE	CALORIES	SLEEP TIME	WAKE UP TIME	WEIGHT
MIN / HRS					

MY ACHIEVEMENTS
☐ _____
☐ _____
☐ _____

How I feel today

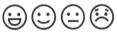

"You can't give up! If you give up, you're like everybody else."
- Chris Evert

DAY **9**

Date_____

MY COMMITMENTS

_____

_____

_____

	BREAKFAST	LUNCH	DINNER	SNACKS
FOOD	_____	_____	_____	_____
	_____	_____	_____	_____
	_____	_____	_____	_____
	_____	_____	_____	_____
	_____	_____	_____	_____
	CALORIES :	CALORIES :	CALORIES :	CALORIES :

WEIGHTS & REPS	FATS	CARBS	PROTEINS

FITNESS	WATER IN TAKE	CALORIES	SLEEP TIME	WAKE UP TIME	WEIGHT
MIN / HRS					

MY ACHIEVEMENTS

☐ _____

☐ _____

☐ _____

How I feel today

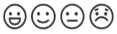

DAY **10**

Date_____

MY COMMITMENTS

_____

_____

_____

FOOD	BREAKFAST	LUNCH	DINNER	SNACKS
	CALORIES :	CALORIES :	CALORIES :	CALORIES :

WEIGHTS & REPS	FATS	CARBS	PROTEINS

FITNESS	WATER IN TAKE	CALORIES	SLEEP TIME	WAKE UP TIME	WEIGHT
MIN / HRS					

MY ACHIEVEMENTS

☐ _____

☐ _____

☐ _____

How I feel today

  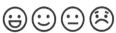

"Step into the new story you are willing to create."
- Oprah Winfrey

DAY **11**

Date_____

MY COMMITMENTS

_____
_____
_____
_____

	BREAKFAST	LUNCH	DINNER	SNACKS
FOOD				
	CALORIES :	CALORIES :	CALORIES :	CALORIES :

WEIGHTS & REPS		FATS	CARBS	PROTEINS

FITNESS	WATER IN TAKE	CALORIES	SLEEP TIME	WAKE UP TIME	WEIGHT
MIN / HRS					

MY ACHIEVEMENTS

☐ _____
☐ _____
☐ _____

How I feel today

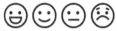

"The question isn't who is going to let me, it's who is going to stop me."
- Ayn Rand

DAY **12**

Date_____

MY COMMITMENTS

_____

_____

_____

FOOD	BREAKFAST	LUNCH	DINNER	SNACKS
	CALORIES :	CALORIES :	CALORIES :	CALORIES :

WEIGHTS & REPS		FATS	CARBS	PROTEINS

FITNESS	WATER IN TAKE	CALORIES	SLEEP TIME	WAKE UP TIME	WEIGHT
MIN / HRS					

MY ACHIEVEMENTS

☐ _____

☐ _____

☐ _____

How I feel today

  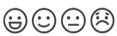

"I learned a long time ago that there is something worse than missing the goal, and that's not pulling the trigger."
- Mia Hamm

DAY **13**

Date_____

MY COMMITMENTS

_____
_____
_____

FOOD	BREAKFAST	LUNCH	DINNER	SNACKS
	_____	_____	_____	_____
	_____	_____	_____	_____
	_____	_____	_____	_____
	_____	_____	_____	_____
	_____	_____	_____	_____
	CALORIES :	CALORIES :	CALORIES :	CALORIES :

WEIGHTS & REPS		FATS	CARBS	PROTEINS

FITNESS	WATER IN TAKE	CALORIES	SLEEP TIME	WAKE UP TIME	WEIGHT
	🥛🥛🥛🥛🥛🥛🥛🥛				
MIN / HRS					

MY ACHIEVEMENTS

☐ _____
☐ _____
☐ _____

How I feel today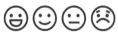

"I do not try to dance better than anyone else.
I only try to dance better than myself."
- Arianna Huffington

DAY **14**

Date_____

MY COMMITMENTS

_____
_____
_____

	BREAKFAST	LUNCH	DINNER	SNACKS
FOOD				
	CALORIES :	CALORIES :	CALORIES :	CALORIES :

WEIGHTS & REPS	FATS	CARBS	PROTEINS

FITNESS	WATER IN TAKE	CALORIES	SLEEP TIME	WAKE UP TIME	WEIGHT
	🥤🥤🥤🥤🥤🥤🥤				
MIN / HRS					

MY ACHIEVEMENTS

☐ _____
☐ _____
☐ _____

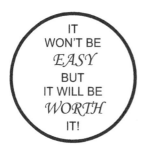

IT
WON'T BE
EASY
BUT
IT WILL BE
WORTH
IT!

WEEKLY CHECK IN

CHECK IN

	M	T	W	T	F	S	S
Drink 8 glasses water	☐	☐	☐	☐	☐	☐	☐
Take my vitamins / supplements	☐	☐	☐	☐	☐	☐	☐
Do my cardio workout	☐	☐	☐	☐	☐	☐	☐
Completed my strength training	☐	☐	☐	☐	☐	☐	☐
Recorded in my food journal	☐	☐	☐	☐	☐	☐	☐
Measured my weight	☐	☐	☐	☐	☐	☐	☐

DID YOU ACCOMPLISH LAST WEEK'S GOALS? IF NOT, WHY?

_____

_____

_____

_____

NEXT WEEK'S GOALS

☐ _____

☐ _____

☐ _____

☐ _____

How I feel today

  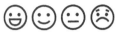

"When I believe in something, I'm like a dog with a bone."
- Melissa McCarthy

DAY **15**

Date_____

MY COMMITMENTS

_____
_____
_____

FOOD	BREAKFAST	LUNCH	DINNER	SNACKS
	_____	_____	_____	_____
	_____	_____	_____	_____
	_____	_____	_____	_____
	_____	_____	_____	_____
	_____	_____	_____	_____
	CALORIES :	CALORIES :	CALORIES :	CALORIES :

WEIGHTS & REPS		FATS	CARBS	PROTEINS

FITNESS	WATER IN TAKE	CALORIES	SLEEP TIME	WAKE UP TIME	WEIGHT
MIN / HRS					

MY ACHIEVEMENTS
☐ _____
☐ _____
☐ _____

How I feel today

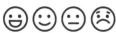

"Without goals, and plans to reach them, you are like a ship that has set sail with no destination."
- Fitzhugh Dodson

DAY **16**

Date_____

MY COMMITMENTS

_____
_____
_____

	BREAKFAST	LUNCH	DINNER	SNACKS
FOOD				
	CALORIES :	CALORIES :	CALORIES :	CALORIES :

WEIGHTS & REPS		FATS	CARBS	PROTEINS

FITNESS	WATER IN TAKE	CALORIES	SLEEP TIME	WAKE UP TIME	WEIGHT
MIN / HRS					

MY ACHIEVEMENTS

- [ ] _____
- [ ] _____
- [ ] _____

How I feel today

  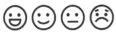

"People with goals succeed because they know where they're going."
- Earl Nightingale

DAY **17**

Date_____

MY COMMITMENTS

_____

_____

_____

FOOD	BREAKFAST	LUNCH	DINNER	SNACKS
	_____	_____	_____	_____
	_____	_____	_____	_____
	_____	_____	_____	_____
	_____	_____	_____	_____
	_____	_____	_____	_____
	CALORIES :	CALORIES :	CALORIES :	CALORIES :

WEIGHTS & REPS		FATS	CARBS	PROTEINS

FITNESS	WATER IN TAKE	CALORIES	SLEEP TIME	WAKE UP TIME	WEIGHT
	🥛🥛🥛🥛🥛🥛🥛				
MIN / HRS					

MY ACHIEVEMENTS

☐ _____

☐ _____

☐ _____

How I feel today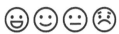

"Obstacles are what you see when you take your eye off the goal."
- Chris Burke

DAY **18**

Date_____

MY COMMITMENTS

_____
_____
_____

FOOD	BREAKFAST	LUNCH	DINNER	SNACKS
	CALORIES :	CALORIES :	CALORIES :	CALORIES :

WEIGHTS & REPS	FATS	CARBS	PROTEINS

FITNESS	WATER IN TAKE	CALORIES	SLEEP TIME	WAKE UP TIME	WEIGHT
	🥛🥛🥛🥛🥛🥛🥛				
MIN / HRS					

MY ACHIEVEMENTS

☐ _____
☐ _____
☐ _____

How I feel today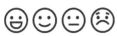

"A year from now you may wish you had started today."
- Karen Lamb

DAY **19**

Date_____

MY COMMITMENTS

_____
_____
_____

FOOD	BREAKFAST	LUNCH	DINNER	SNACKS
	_____	_____	_____	_____
	_____	_____	_____	_____
	_____	_____	_____	_____
	_____	_____	_____	_____
	_____	_____	_____	_____
	CALORIES :	CALORIES :	CALORIES :	CALORIES :

WEIGHTS & REPS	FATS	CARBS	PROTEINS

FITNESS	WATER IN TAKE	CALORIES	SLEEP TIME	WAKE UP TIME	WEIGHT
MIN / HRS					

MY ACHIEVEMENTS

- ☐ _____
- ☐ _____
- ☐ _____

How I feel today

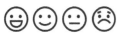

"When defeat comes, accept it as a signal that your plans are not sound, rebuild those plans, and set sail once more toward your coveted goal."
- Napoleon Hill

DAY **20**

Date_____

MY COMMITMENTS

_____

_____

_____

FOOD	BREAKFAST	LUNCH	DINNER	SNACKS
	CALORIES :	CALORIES :	CALORIES :	CALORIES :

WEIGHTS & REPS	FATS	CARBS	PROTEINS

FITNESS	WATER IN TAKE	CALORIES	SLEEP TIME	WAKE UP TIME	WEIGHT
MIN / HRS					

MY ACHIEVEMENTS

☐ _____

☐ _____

☐ _____

How I feel today

😃 ☺ 😐 ☹

DAY **21**

Date_____

MY COMMITMENTS

_____
_____
_____

	BREAKFAST	LUNCH	DINNER	SNACKS
FOOD	_____ _____ _____ _____ _____	_____ _____ _____ _____ _____	_____ _____ _____ _____ _____	_____ _____ _____ _____ _____
	CALORIES :	CALORIES :	CALORIES :	CALORIES :

WEIGHTS & REPS		FATS	CARBS	PROTEINS

FITNESS	WATER IN TAKE	CALORIES	SLEEP TIME	WAKE UP TIME	WEIGHT
	🥛🥛🥛🥛🥛🥛🥛				
MIN / HRS					

MY ACHIEVEMENTS
☐ _____
☐ _____
☐ _____

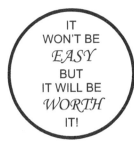

IT WON'T BE *EASY* BUT IT WILL BE *WORTH* IT!

WEEKLY CHECK IN

CHECK IN

	M	T	W	T	F	S	S
Drink 8 glasses water	☐	☐	☐	☐	☐	☐	☐
Take my vitamins / supplements	☐	☐	☐	☐	☐	☐	☐
Do my cardio workout	☐	☐	☐	☐	☐	☐	☐
Completed my strength training	☐	☐	☐	☐	☐	☐	☐
Recorded in my food journal	☐	☐	☐	☐	☐	☐	☐
Measured my weight	☐	☐	☐	☐	☐	☐	☐
	☐	☐	☐	☐	☐	☐	☐

DID YOU ACCOMPLISH LAST WEEK'S GOALS? IF NOT, WHY?

_____

_____

_____

_____

NEXT WEEK'S GOALS

☐ _____

☐ _____

☐ _____

☐ _____

How I feel today

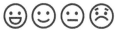

"I can't change the direction of the wind, but I can adjust my sails to always reach my destination."
- Jimmy Dean

DAY **22**

Date_____

MY COMMITMENTS

_____

_____

_____

FOOD	BREAKFAST	LUNCH	DINNER	SNACKS
	CALORIES :	CALORIES :	CALORIES :	CALORIES :

WEIGHTS & REPS	FATS	CARBS	PROTEINS

FITNESS	WATER IN TAKE	CALORIES	SLEEP TIME	WAKE UP TIME	WEIGHT
MIN / HRS	🥛🥛🥛🥛🥛🥛🥛🥛				

MY ACHIEVEMENTS

☐ _____

☐ _____

☐ _____

How I feel today

  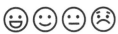

*"You can, you should,
and if you're brave enough to start,
you will."*
- Stephen King

DAY **23**

Date_____

<u>MY COMMITMENTS</u>

_____
_____
_____

FOOD	BREAKFAST	LUNCH	DINNER	SNACKS
	_____	_____	_____	_____
	_____	_____	_____	_____
	_____	_____	_____	_____
	_____	_____	_____	_____
	_____	_____	_____	_____
	CALORIES :	CALORIES :	CALORIES :	CALORIES :

WEIGHTS & REPS		FATS	CARBS	PROTEINS

FITNESS	WATER IN TAKE	CALORIES	SLEEP TIME	WAKE UP TIME	WEIGHT
	🥤🥤🥤🥤🥤🥤🥤				
MIN / HRS					

MY ACHIEVEMENTS

☐ _____
☐ _____
☐ _____

How I feel today

"If a goal is worth having, it's worth blocking out the time in your day-to-day life necessary to achieve it."
- Jill Koenig

DAY **24**

Date_____

MY COMMITMENTS

_____
_____
_____

FOOD	BREAKFAST	LUNCH	DINNER	SNACKS
	CALORIES :	CALORIES :	CALORIES :	CALORIES :

WEIGHTS & REPS	FATS	CARBS	PROTEINS

FITNESS	WATER IN TAKE	CALORIES	SLEEP TIME	WAKE UP TIME	WEIGHT
MIN / HRS					

MY ACHIEVEMENTS

☐ _____
☐ _____
☐ _____

How I feel today

"You don't have to be a fantastic hero.
You can be just an ordinary chap,
motivated to reach challenging goals."
- Edmund Hillary

DAY **25**

Date_____

MY COMMITMENTS

FOOD	BREAKFAST	LUNCH	DINNER	SNACKS
	CALORIES :	CALORIES :	CALORIES :	CALORIES :

WEIGHTS & REPS		FATS	CARBS	PROTEINS

FITNESS	WATER IN TAKE	CALORIES	SLEEP TIME	WAKE UP TIME	WEIGHT
MIN / HRS					

MY ACHIEVEMENTS

- ☐
- ☐
- ☐

How I feel today

DAY **26**

Date_____

MY COMMITMENTS

_____

_____

_____

FOOD	BREAKFAST	LUNCH	DINNER	SNACKS
	_____	_____	_____	_____
	_____	_____	_____	_____
	_____	_____	_____	_____
	_____	_____	_____	_____
	_____	_____	_____	_____
	CALORIES :	CALORIES :	CALORIES :	CALORIES :

WEIGHTS & REPS		FATS	CARBS	PROTEINS

FITNESS	WATER IN TAKE	CALORIES	SLEEP TIME	WAKE UP TIME	WEIGHT
MIN / HRS					

MY ACHIEVEMENTS

- ☐ _____
- ☐ _____
- ☐ _____

How I feel today

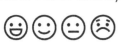

"You can't catch a fish unless you put your line in the water.
You can't reach your goals if you don't try."
- Kathy Seligman

DAY **27**

Date_____

<u>MY COMMITMENTS</u>

_____
_____
_____

FOOD	BREAKFAST	LUNCH	DINNER	SNACKS
	_____	_____	_____	_____
	_____	_____	_____	_____
	_____	_____	_____	_____
	_____	_____	_____	_____
	_____	_____	_____	_____
	CALORIES :	CALORIES :	CALORIES :	CALORIES :

WEIGHTS & REPS		FATS	CARBS	PROTEINS

FITNESS	WATER IN TAKE	CALORIES	SLEEP TIME	WAKE UP TIME	WEIGHT
MIN / HRS					

MY ACHIEVEMENTS

☐ _____
☐ _____
☐

How I feel today

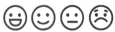

"Obstacles can't stop you. Problems can't stop you. Most of all, other people can't stop you. Only you can stop you."
- Amelia Earhart

DAY **28**

Date_____

MY COMMITMENTS

_____

_____

_____

FOOD	BREAKFAST	LUNCH	DINNER	SNACKS
	_____	_____	_____	_____
	_____	_____	_____	_____
	_____	_____	_____	_____
	_____	_____	_____	_____
	_____	_____	_____	_____
	CALORIES :	CALORIES :	CALORIES :	CALORIES :

WEIGHTS & REPS		FATS	CARBS	PROTEINS

FITNESS	WATER IN TAKE	CALORIES	SLEEP TIME	WAKE UP TIME	WEIGHT
MIN / HRS					

MY ACHIEVEMENTS

☐ _____

☐ _____

☐ _____

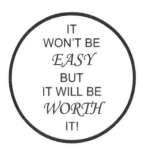

IT
WON'T BE
EASY
BUT
IT WILL BE
WORTH
IT!

WEEKLY CHECK IN

CHECK IN

	M	T	W	T	F	S	S
Drink 8 glasses water	☐	☐	☐	☐	☐	☐	☐
Take my vitamins / supplements	☐	☐	☐	☐	☐	☐	☐
Do my cardio workout	☐	☐	☐	☐	☐	☐	☐
Completed my strength training	☐	☐	☐	☐	☐	☐	☐
Recorded in my food journal	☐	☐	☐	☐	☐	☐	☐
Measured my weight	☐	☐	☐	☐	☐	☐	☐
	☐	☐	☐	☐	☐	☐	☐

DID YOU ACCOMPLISH LAST WEEK'S GOALS? IF NOT, WHY?

_____

_____

_____

_____

NEXT WEEK'S GOALS

☐ _____

☐ _____

☐ _____

☐ _____

How I feel today

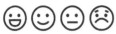

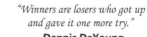

"Winners are losers who got up and gave it one more try."
- **Dennis DeYoung**

DAY **29**

Date_____

MY COMMITMENTS

_____

_____

_____

FOOD	BREAKFAST	LUNCH	DINNER	SNACKS
	_____	_____	_____	_____
	_____	_____	_____	_____
	_____	_____	_____	_____
	_____	_____	_____	_____
	_____	_____	_____	_____
	CALORIES :	CALORIES :	CALORIES :	CALORIES :

WEIGHTS & REPS		FATS	CARBS	PROTEINS

FITNESS	WATER IN TAKE	CALORIES	SLEEP TIME	WAKE UP TIME	WEIGHT
	🥛🥛🥛🥛🥛🥛🥛🥛				
MIN / HRS					

MY ACHIEVEMENTS

☐ _____

☐ _____

☐ _____

How I feel today

"If you want to be happy,
set a goal that commands your thoughts,
liberates your energy and inspires your hopes."
- Andrew Carnegie

DAY **30**

Date_____

MY COMMITMENTS

_____

_____

_____

FOOD	BREAKFAST	LUNCH	DINNER	SNACKS
	CALORIES :	CALORIES :	CALORIES :	CALORIES :

WEIGHTS & REPS	FATS	CARBS	PROTEINS

FITNESS	WATER IN TAKE	CALORIES	SLEEP TIME	WAKE UP TIME	WEIGHT
MIN / HRS	🥛🥛🥛🥛🥛🥛🥛				

MY ACHIEVEMENTS

☐ _____

☐ _____

☐ _____

How I feel today

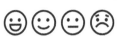

"A dream becomes a goal when action is taken toward its achievement."
- Bo Bennett

Date_____

MY COMMITMENTS

_____

_____

_____

FOOD	BREAKFAST	LUNCH	DINNER	SNACKS
	_____	_____	_____	_____
	_____	_____	_____	_____
	_____	_____	_____	_____
	_____	_____	_____	_____
	_____	_____	_____	_____
	CALORIES :	CALORIES :	CALORIES :	CALORIES :

WEIGHTS & REPS		FATS	CARBS	PROTEINS

FITNESS	WATER IN TAKE	CALORIES	SLEEP TIME	WAKE UP TIME	WEIGHT
MIN / HRS					

MY ACHIEVEMENTS

☐ _____

☐ _____

☐ _____

How I feel today

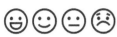

"God gives us dreams a size too big so that we can grow into them."
- Unknown

DAY **32**

Date_____

MY COMMITMENTS

_____
_____
_____

	BREAKFAST	LUNCH	DINNER	SNACKS
FOOD	_____ _____ _____ _____ _____	_____ _____ _____ _____ _____	_____ _____ _____ _____ _____	_____ _____ _____ _____ _____
	CALORIES :	CALORIES :	CALORIES :	CALORIES :

WEIGHTS & REPS		FATS	CARBS	PROTEINS

FITNESS	WATER IN TAKE	CALORIES	SLEEP TIME	WAKE UP TIME	WEIGHT
MIN / HRS					

MY ACHIEVEMENTS

☐ _____
☐ _____
☐ _____

How I feel today

"One part at a time, one day at a time, we can accomplish any goal we set for ourselves."
- Karen Casey

_____ DAY **33**

Date_____

MY COMMITMENTS

_____
_____
_____

FOOD	BREAKFAST	LUNCH	DINNER	SNACKS
	_____	_____	_____	_____
	_____	_____	_____	_____
	_____	_____	_____	_____
	_____	_____	_____	_____
	_____	_____	_____	_____
	CALORIES :	CALORIES :	CALORIES :	CALORIES :

WEIGHTS & REPS		FATS	CARBS	PROTEINS

FITNESS	WATER IN TAKE	CALORIES	SLEEP TIME	WAKE UP TIME	WEIGHT
MIN / HRS					

MY ACHIEVEMENTS

☐ _____
☐ _____
☐ _____

How I feel today *"It doesn't matter where you are coming from. All that matters is where you are going."* **- Brian Tracy**

DAY **34**

Date_____

MY COMMITMENTS

_____
_____
_____

FOOD	BREAKFAST	LUNCH	DINNER	SNACKS
	_____	_____	_____	_____
	_____	_____	_____	_____
	_____	_____	_____	_____
	_____	_____	_____	_____
	_____	_____	_____	_____
	CALORIES :	CALORIES :	CALORIES :	CALORIES :

WEIGHTS & REPS	FATS	CARBS	PROTEINS

FITNESS	WATER IN TAKE	CALORIES	SLEEP TIME	WAKE UP TIME	WEIGHT
MIN / HRS					

MY ACHIEVEMENTS
☐ _____
☐ _____
☐ _____

How I feel today

"Do not let what you cannot do interfere with what you can do."
- John Wooden

DAY **35**

Date_____

MY COMMITMENTS

_____
_____
_____

	BREAKFAST	LUNCH	DINNER	SNACKS
FOOD	_____	_____	_____	_____
	_____	_____	_____	_____
	_____	_____	_____	_____
	_____	_____	_____	_____
	_____	_____	_____	_____
	CALORIES :	CALORIES :	CALORIES :	CALORIES :

WEIGHTS & REPS		FATS	CARBS	PROTEINS

FITNESS	WATER IN TAKE	CALORIES	SLEEP TIME	WAKE UP TIME	WEIGHT
	🥛🥛🥛🥛🥛🥛🥛				
MIN / HRS					

MY ACHIEVEMENTS

☐ _____
☐ _____
☐ _____

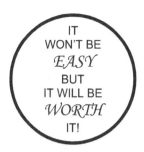

IT
WON'T BE
EASY
BUT
IT WILL BE
WORTH
IT!

WEEKLY CHECK IN

CHECK IN

	M	T	W	T	F	S	S
Drink 8 glasses water	☐	☐	☐	☐	☐	☐	☐
Take my vitamins / supplements	☐	☐	☐	☐	☐	☐	☐
Do my cardio workout	☐	☐	☐	☐	☐	☐	☐
Completed my strength training	☐	☐	☐	☐	☐	☐	☐
Recorded in my food journal	☐	☐	☐	☐	☐	☐	☐
Measured my weight	☐	☐	☐	☐	☐	☐	☐

DID YOU ACCOMPLISH LAST WEEK'S GOALS? IF NOT, WHY?

_____

_____

_____

_____

NEXT WEEK'S GOALS

☐ _____

☐ _____

☐ _____

☐ _____

How I feel today

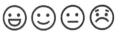

"Discipline is the bridge between goals and accomplishment."
- Jim Rohn

DAY **36**

Date_____

MY COMMITMENTS

_____

_____

_____

FOOD	BREAKFAST	LUNCH	DINNER	SNACKS
	_____	_____	_____	_____
	_____	_____	_____	_____
	_____	_____	_____	_____
	_____	_____	_____	_____
	_____	_____	_____	_____
	CALORIES :	CALORIES :	CALORIES :	CALORIES :

WEIGHTS & REPS		FATS	CARBS	PROTEINS

FITNESS	WATER IN TAKE	CALORIES	SLEEP TIME	WAKE UP TIME	WEIGHT
	🥛🥛🥛🥛🥛🥛🥛				
MIN / HRS					

MY ACHIEVEMENTS
☐ _____
☐ _____
☐ _____

How I feel today

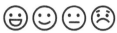

"Begin with the end in mind."
- Stephen Covey

_____ DAY **37**

Date_____

MY COMMITMENTS

_____

_____

_____

FOOD	BREAKFAST	LUNCH	DINNER	SNACKS
	_____	_____	_____	_____
	_____	_____	_____	_____
	_____	_____	_____	_____
	_____	_____	_____	_____
	_____	_____	_____	_____
	CALORIES :	CALORIES :	CALORIES :	CALORIES :

WEIGHTS & REPS		FATS	CARBS	PROTEINS

FITNESS	WATER IN TAKE	CALORIES	SLEEP TIME	WAKE UP TIME	WEIGHT
	🥛🥛🥛🥛🥛🥛🥛				
MIN / HRS					

MY ACHIEVEMENTS
☐ _____
☐ _____
☐ _____

How I feel today

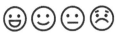

"You miss 100 percent of the shots you don't take."
- Wayne Gretsky

DAY **38**

Date_____

MY COMMITMENTS

_____

_____

_____

FOOD	BREAKFAST	LUNCH	DINNER	SNACKS
	_____	_____	_____	_____
	_____	_____	_____	_____
	_____	_____	_____	_____
	_____	_____	_____	_____
	_____	_____	_____	_____
	CALORIES :	CALORIES :	CALORIES :	CALORIES :

WEIGHTS & REPS		FATS	CARBS	PROTEINS

FITNESS	WATER IN TAKE	CALORIES	SLEEP TIME	WAKE UP TIME	WEIGHT
	🥛🥛🥛🥛🥛🥛🥛				
MIN / HRS					

MY ACHIEVEMENTS

☐ _____

☐ _____

☐ _____

How I feel today

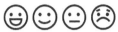

"Believe you can and you're halfway there."
- Theodore Roosevelt

_____ DAY **39**

Date_____

MY COMMITMENTS

_____
_____
_____

FOOD	BREAKFAST	LUNCH	DINNER	SNACKS
	CALORIES :	CALORIES :	CALORIES :	CALORIES :

WEIGHTS & REPS		FATS	CARBS	PROTEINS

FITNESS	WATER IN TAKE	CALORIES	SLEEP TIME	WAKE UP TIME	WEIGHT
MIN / HRS					

MY ACHIEVEMENTS

☐ _____
☐ _____
☐ _____

How I feel today

"When you know what you want and you want it bad enough, you'll find a way to get it."
- Jim Rohn

DAY **40**

Date_____

MY COMMITMENTS

_____

_____

_____

FOOD	BREAKFAST	LUNCH	DINNER	SNACKS
	_____	_____	_____	_____
	_____	_____	_____	_____
	_____	_____	_____	_____
	_____	_____	_____	_____
	_____	_____	_____	_____
	CALORIES :	CALORIES :	CALORIES :	CALORIES :

WEIGHTS & REPS		FATS	CARBS	PROTEINS

FITNESS	WATER IN TAKE	CALORIES	SLEEP TIME	WAKE UP TIME	WEIGHT
MIN / HRS	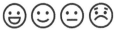				

MY ACHIEVEMENTS

☐ _____

☐ _____

☐ _____

How I feel today

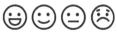

"Decide whether or not the goal is worth the risks involved. If it is, stop worrying."
- Amelia Earhart

DAY **41**

Date_____

MY COMMITMENTS

_____

_____

_____

FOOD	BREAKFAST	LUNCH	DINNER	SNACKS
	_____	_____	_____	_____
	_____	_____	_____	_____
	_____	_____	_____	_____
	_____	_____	_____	_____
	_____	_____	_____	_____
	CALORIES :	CALORIES :	CALORIES :	CALORIES :

WEIGHTS & REPS		FATS	CARBS	PROTEINS

FITNESS	WATER IN TAKE	CALORIES	SLEEP TIME	WAKE UP TIME	WEIGHT
MIN / HRS	🥛🥛🥛🥛🥛🥛🥛🥛				

MY ACHIEVEMENTS
☐ _____
☐ _____
☐ _____

How I feel today

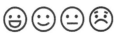

DAY **42**

Date_____

MY COMMITMENTS

_____
_____
_____

FOOD	BREAKFAST	LUNCH	DINNER	SNACKS
	_____	_____	_____	_____
	_____	_____	_____	_____
	_____	_____	_____	_____
	_____	_____	_____	_____
	_____	_____	_____	_____
	CALORIES :	CALORIES :	CALORIES :	CALORIES :

WEIGHTS & REPS	FATS	CARBS	PROTEINS

FITNESS	WATER IN TAKE	CALORIES	SLEEP TIME	WAKE UP TIME	WEIGHT
MIN / HRS					

MY ACHIEVEMENTS

- ☐ _____
- ☐ _____
- ☐ _____

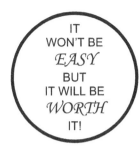

IT
WON'T BE
EASY
BUT
IT WILL BE
WORTH
IT!

WEEKLY CHECK IN

CHECK IN

	M	T	W	T	F	S	S
Drink 8 glasses water	☐	☐	☐	☐	☐	☐	☐
Take my vitamins / supplements	☐	☐	☐	☐	☐	☐	☐
Do my cardio workout	☐	☐	☐	☐	☐	☐	☐
Completed my strength training	☐	☐	☐	☐	☐	☐	☐
Recorded in my food journal	☐	☐	☐	☐	☐	☐	☐
Measured my weight	☐	☐	☐	☐	☐	☐	☐

DID YOU ACCOMPLISH LAST WEEK'S GOALS? IF NOT, WHY?

_____

_____

_____

_____

NEXT WEEK'S GOALS

☐ _____

☐ _____

☐ _____

☐ _____

How I feel today

  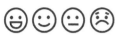

"Set remarkable goals for yourself and get to work on achieving them. Then, watch in amazement as you become remarkable."
- Marelisa Fabrega

DAY **43**

Date_____

MY COMMITMENTS

_____
_____
_____

	BREAKFAST	LUNCH	DINNER	SNACKS
FOOD				
	CALORIES :	CALORIES :	CALORIES :	CALORIES :

WEIGHTS & REPS		FATS	CARBS	PROTEINS

FITNESS	WATER IN TAKE	CALORIES	SLEEP TIME	WAKE UP TIME	WEIGHT
MIN / HRS					

MY ACHIEVEMENTS
☐ _____
☐ _____
☐ _____

How I feel today

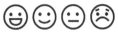

"It Is Never Too Late To Be What You Might Have Been."
- Anonymous

DAY **44**

Date_____

MY COMMITMENTS

_____
_____
_____

FOOD	BREAKFAST	LUNCH	DINNER	SNACKS
	_____	_____	_____	_____
	_____	_____	_____	_____
	_____	_____	_____	_____
	_____	_____	_____	_____
	_____	_____	_____	_____
	CALORIES :	CALORIES :	CALORIES :	CALORIES :

WEIGHTS & REPS		FATS	CARBS	PROTEINS

FITNESS	WATER IN TAKE	CALORIES	SLEEP TIME	WAKE UP TIME	WEIGHT
MIN / HRS					

MY ACHIEVEMENTS

☐ _____
☐ _____
☐ _____

How I feel today

😀 🙂 😐 ☹️

"Do what you have to do until you can do what you want to do."
- Oprah Winfrey

DAY **45**

Date_____

MY COMMITMENTS

_____
_____
_____

FOOD	BREAKFAST	LUNCH	DINNER	SNACKS
	CALORIES :	CALORIES :	CALORIES :	CALORIES :

WEIGHTS & REPS		FATS	CARBS	PROTEINS

FITNESS	WATER IN TAKE	CALORIES	SLEEP TIME	WAKE UP TIME	WEIGHT
	🥛🥛🥛🥛🥛🥛🥛🥛				
MIN / HRS					

MY ACHIEVEMENTS

☐ _____
☐ _____
☐ _____

How I feel today

😄 😊 😐 😦

*"Set your goals high,
and don't stop until you get there."*
- Bo Jackson

DAY **46**

Date_____

MY COMMITMENTS

_____
_____
_____

FOOD	BREAKFAST	LUNCH	DINNER	SNACKS
	CALORIES :	CALORIES :	CALORIES :	CALORIES :

WEIGHTS & REPS		FATS	CARBS	PROTEINS

FITNESS	WATER IN TAKE	CALORIES	SLEEP TIME	WAKE UP TIME	WEIGHT
	🥛🥛🥛🥛🥛🥛🥛🥛				
MIN / HRS					

MY ACHIEVEMENTS

☐ _____
☐ _____
☐ _____

How I feel today

"Setting goals is the first step in turning the invisible into the visible."
- Tony Robbins

DAY **47**

Date_____

MY COMMITMENTS

_____

_____

_____

FOOD	BREAKFAST	LUNCH	DINNER	SNACKS
	CALORIES :	CALORIES :	CALORIES :	CALORIES :

WEIGHTS & REPS		FATS	CARBS	PROTEINS

FITNESS	WATER IN TAKE	CALORIES	SLEEP TIME	WAKE UP TIME	WEIGHT
	🥃🥃🥃🥃🥃🥃🥃				
MIN / HRS					

MY ACHIEVEMENTS
☐ _____
☐ _____
☐ _____

How I feel today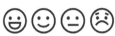

"What you get by achieving your goals is not as important as what you become by achieving your goals."
- Zig Ziglar

DAY **48**

Date_____

MY COMMITMENTS

_____
_____
_____
_____

FOOD	BREAKFAST	LUNCH	DINNER	SNACKS
	CALORIES :	CALORIES :	CALORIES :	CALORIES :

WEIGHTS & REPS	FATS	CARBS	PROTEINS

FITNESS	WATER IN TAKE	CALORIES	SLEEP TIME	WAKE UP TIME	WEIGHT
MIN / HRS					

MY ACHIEVEMENTS

☐ _____
☐ _____
☐ _____

How I feel today

😆 🙂 😐 😖

DAY **49**

Date_____

MY COMMITMENTS

_____
_____
_____

FOOD	BREAKFAST	LUNCH	DINNER	SNACKS
	_____	_____	_____	_____
	_____	_____	_____	_____
	_____	_____	_____	_____
	_____	_____	_____	_____
	_____	_____	_____	_____
	CALORIES :	CALORIES :	CALORIES :	CALORIES :

WEIGHTS & REPS		FATS	CARBS	PROTEINS

FITNESS	WATER IN TAKE	CALORIES	SLEEP TIME	WAKE UP TIME	WEIGHT
	🥛🥛🥛🥛🥛🥛🥛				
MIN / HRS					

MY ACHIEVEMENTS

☐ _____
☐ _____
☐ _____

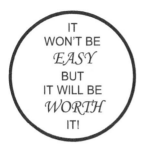

IT WON'T BE *EASY* BUT IT WILL BE *WORTH* IT!

WEEKLY
CHECK IN

CHECK IN

	M	T	W	T	F	S	S
Drink 8 glasses water	☐	☐	☐	☐	☐	☐	☐
Take my vitamins / supplements	☐	☐	☐	☐	☐	☐	☐
Do my cardio workout	☐	☐	☐	☐	☐	☐	☐
Completed my strength training	☐	☐	☐	☐	☐	☐	☐
Recorded in my food journal	☐	☐	☐	☐	☐	☐	☐
Measured my weight	☐	☐	☐	☐	☐	☐	☐
	☐	☐	☐	☐	☐	☐	☐

DID YOU ACCOMPLISH LAST WEEK'S GOALS? IF NOT, WHY?

_____

_____

_____

_____

NEXT WEEK'S GOALS

☐ _____

☐ _____

☐ _____

☐ _____

How I feel today

"One way to keep momentum going is to have constantly greater goals."
- Michael Korda

DAY **50**

Date_____

MY COMMITMENTS

_____

_____

_____

FOOD	BREAKFAST	LUNCH	DINNER	SNACKS
	_____	_____	_____	_____
	_____	_____	_____	_____
	_____	_____	_____	_____
	_____	_____	_____	_____
	_____	_____	_____	_____
	CALORIES :	CALORIES :	CALORIES :	CALORIES :

WEIGHTS & REPS		FATS	CARBS	PROTEINS

FITNESS	WATER IN TAKE	CALORIES	SLEEP TIME	WAKE UP TIME	WEIGHT
MIN / HRS	🥛🥛🥛🥛🥛🥛🥛🥛				

MY ACHIEVEMENTS

☐ _____

☐ _____

☐ _____

How I feel today

"People with goals succeed because they know where they're going."
- Earl Nightingale

DAY **51**

Date_____

MY COMMITMENTS

_____

_____

_____

FOOD	BREAKFAST	LUNCH	DINNER	SNACKS
	_____	_____	_____	_____
	_____	_____	_____	_____
	_____	_____	_____	_____
	_____	_____	_____	_____
	_____	_____	_____	_____
	CALORIES :	CALORIES :	CALORIES :	CALORIES :

WEIGHTS & REPS			FATS	CARBS	PROTEINS

FITNESS	WATER IN TAKE	CALORIES	SLEEP TIME	WAKE UP TIME	WEIGHT
	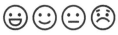				
MIN / HRS					

MY ACHIEVEMENTS

☐ _____

☐ _____

☐ _____

How I feel today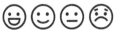

"You need to overcome the tug of people against you as you reach for high goals."
- George S. Patton

DAY **52**

Date_____

MY COMMITMENTS

_____

_____

_____

FOOD	BREAKFAST	LUNCH	DINNER	SNACKS
	CALORIES :	CALORIES :	CALORIES :	CALORIES :

WEIGHTS & REPS		FATS	CARBS	PROTEINS

FITNESS	WATER IN TAKE	CALORIES	SLEEP TIME	WAKE UP TIME	WEIGHT
MIN / HRS					

MY ACHIEVEMENTS
☐ _____
☐ _____
☐ _____

How I feel today

"Success is steady progress toward one's personal goals."
- Jim Rohn

DAY **53**

Date_____

MY COMMITMENTS

_____
_____
_____
_____

	BREAKFAST	LUNCH	DINNER	SNACKS
FOOD	_____ _____ _____ _____ _____	_____ _____ _____ _____ _____	_____ _____ _____ _____ _____	_____ _____ _____ _____ _____
	CALORIES :	CALORIES :	CALORIES :	CALORIES :

WEIGHTS & REPS		FATS	CARBS	PROTEINS

FITNESS	WATER IN TAKE	CALORIES	SLEEP TIME	WAKE UP TIME	WEIGHT
MIN / HRS					

MY ACHIEVEMENTS
☐ _____
☐ _____
☐ _____

How I feel today

"Goals transform a random walk into a chase."
- Mihaly Csikszentmihalyi

DAY **54**

Date_____

MY COMMITMENTS

_____

_____

_____

FOOD	BREAKFAST	LUNCH	DINNER	SNACKS
	_____	_____	_____	_____
	_____	_____	_____	_____
	_____	_____	_____	_____
	_____	_____	_____	_____
	_____	_____	_____	_____
	CALORIES :	CALORIES :	CALORIES :	CALORIES :

WEIGHTS & REPS	FATS	CARBS	PROTEINS

FITNESS	WATER IN TAKE	CALORIES	SLEEP TIME	WAKE UP TIME	WEIGHT
MIN / HRS	🥤🥤🥤🥤🥤🥤🥤				

MY ACHIEVEMENTS
☐ _____
☐ _____
☐ _____

How I feel today

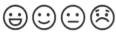

"No matter how many goals you have achieved, you must set your sights on a higher one."
- Jessica Savitch

DAY **55**

Date_____

MY COMMITMENTS

_____
_____
_____

FOOD	BREAKFAST	LUNCH	DINNER	SNACKS
	_____	_____	_____	_____
	_____	_____	_____	_____
	_____	_____	_____	_____
	_____	_____	_____	_____
	_____	_____	_____	_____
	CALORIES :	CALORIES :	CALORIES :	CALORIES :

WEIGHTS & REPS		FATS	CARBS	PROTEINS

FITNESS	WATER IN TAKE	CALORIES	SLEEP TIME	WAKE UP TIME	WEIGHT
MIN / HRS	🥛🥛🥛🥛🥛🥛🥛🥛				

MY ACHIEVEMENTS

☐ _____
☐ _____
☐ _____

How I feel today

 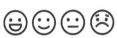

"You must take action now
that will move you towards your goals."
- H. Jackson Brown, Jr.

DAY **56**

Date_____

MY COMMITMENTS

_____
_____
_____

	BREAKFAST	LUNCH	DINNER	SNACKS
FOOD	_____	_____	_____	_____
	CALORIES :	CALORIES :	CALORIES :	CALORIES :

WEIGHTS & REPS		FATS	CARBS	PROTEINS

FITNESS	WATER IN TAKE	CALORIES	SLEEP TIME	WAKE UP TIME	WEIGHT
	🥛🥛🥛🥛🥛🥛🥛				
MIN / HRS					

MY ACHIEVEMENTS

☐ _____
☐ _____
☐ _____

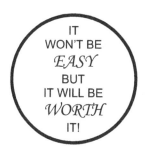

IT
WON'T BE
EASY
BUT
IT WILL BE
WORTH
IT!

WEEKLY CHECK IN

CHECK IN

	M	T	W	T	F	S	S
Drink 8 glasses water	☐	☐	☐	☐	☐	☐	☐
Take my vitamins / supplements	☐	☐	☐	☐	☐	☐	☐
Do my cardio workout	☐	☐	☐	☐	☐	☐	☐
Completed my strength training	☐	☐	☐	☐	☐	☐	☐
Recorded in my food journal	☐	☐	☐	☐	☐	☐	☐
Measured my weight	☐	☐	☐	☐	☐	☐	☐
	☐	☐	☐	☐	☐	☐	☐

DID YOU ACCOMPLISH LAST WEEK'S GOALS? IF NOT, WHY?

_____

_____

_____

_____

NEXT WEEK'S GOALS

☐ _____

☐ _____

☐ _____

☐ _____

How I feel today

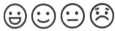

"You must be passionate, you must dedicate yourself, and you must be relentless in the pursuit of your goals."
- Steve Garvey

DAY **57**

Date_____

MY COMMITMENTS

_____
_____
_____

FOOD	BREAKFAST	LUNCH	DINNER	SNACKS
	_____	_____	_____	_____
	_____	_____	_____	_____
	_____	_____	_____	_____
	_____	_____	_____	_____
	_____	_____	_____	_____
	CALORIES :	CALORIES :	CALORIES :	CALORIES :

WEIGHTS & REPS		FATS	CARBS	PROTEINS

FITNESS	WATER IN TAKE	CALORIES	SLEEP TIME	WAKE UP TIME	WEIGHT
MIN / HRS					

MY ACHIEVEMENTS

☐ _____
☐ _____
☐ _____

How I feel today

"I Am Not What Happened To Me.
I Am What I Choose To Become."
- Anonymous

DAY **58**

Date_____

MY COMMITMENTS

_____
_____
_____
_____

FOOD	BREAKFAST	LUNCH	DINNER	SNACKS
	_____	_____	_____	_____
	_____	_____	_____	_____
	_____	_____	_____	_____
	_____	_____	_____	_____
	_____	_____	_____	_____
	CALORIES :	CALORIES :	CALORIES :	CALORIES :

WEIGHTS & REPS		FATS	CARBS	PROTEINS

FITNESS	WATER IN TAKE	CALORIES	SLEEP TIME	WAKE UP TIME	WEIGHT
	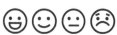				
MIN / HRS					

MY ACHIEVEMENTS

☐ _____
☐ _____
☐ _____

How I feel today

  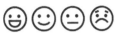

"It Always Seems Impossible Until It's Done."
- Anonymous

DAY **59**

Date_____

MY COMMITMENTS

_____

_____

_____

FOOD	BREAKFAST	LUNCH	DINNER	SNACKS
	_____	_____	_____	_____
	_____	_____	_____	_____
	_____	_____	_____	_____
	_____	_____	_____	_____
	_____	_____	_____	_____
	CALORIES :	CALORIES :	CALORIES :	CALORIES :

WEIGHTS & REPS		FATS	CARBS	PROTEINS

FITNESS	WATER IN TAKE	CALORIES	SLEEP TIME	WAKE UP TIME	WEIGHT
MIN / HRS					

MY ACHIEVEMENTS

☐ _____
☐ _____
☐ _____

How I feel today

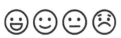

"Fall Seven Times, Stand Up Eight ."
- Anonymous

DAY **60**

Date_____

MY COMMITMENTS

_____

_____

_____

FOOD	BREAKFAST	LUNCH	DINNER	SNACKS
	CALORIES :	CALORIES :	CALORIES :	CALORIES :

WEIGHTS & REPS		FATS	CARBS	PROTEINS

FITNESS	WATER IN TAKE	CALORIES	SLEEP TIME	WAKE UP TIME	WEIGHT
	🥛🥛🥛🥛🥛🥛🥛				
MIN / HRS					

MY ACHIEVEMENTS

☐ _____

☐ _____

☐ _____

How I feel today

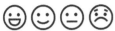

"The height of my goals will not hold me in awe, though I may stumble often before they are reached."
- Og Mandino

DAY **61**

Date_____

MY COMMITMENTS

_____

_____

_____

FOOD	BREAKFAST	LUNCH	DINNER	SNACKS
	_____	_____	_____	_____
	_____	_____	_____	_____
	_____	_____	_____	_____
	_____	_____	_____	_____
	_____	_____	_____	_____
	CALORIES :	CALORIES :	CALORIES :	CALORIES :

WEIGHTS & REPS		FATS	CARBS	PROTEINS

FITNESS	WATER IN TAKE	CALORIES	SLEEP TIME	WAKE UP TIME	WEIGHT
	🥤🥤🥤🥤🥤🥤🥤				
MIN / HRS					

MY ACHIEVEMENTS

☐ _____

☐ _____

☐ _____

How I feel today

DAY **62**

Date_____

MY COMMITMENTS

_____

_____

_____

FOOD	BREAKFAST	LUNCH	DINNER	SNACKS
	CALORIES :	CALORIES :	CALORIES :	CALORIES :

WEIGHTS & REPS		FATS	CARBS	PROTEINS

FITNESS	WATER IN TAKE	CALORIES	SLEEP TIME	WAKE UP TIME	WEIGHT
	🥛🥛🥛🥛🥛🥛🥛🥛				
MIN / HRS					

MY ACHIEVEMENTS

☐ _____

☐ _____

☐ _____

How I feel today

"You've only got 3 choices in life: Give up, give in, or give it all you've got."
- Anonymous

DAY **63**

Date_____

MY COMMITMENTS

_____
_____
_____

FOOD	BREAKFAST	LUNCH	DINNER	SNACKS
	_____	_____	_____	_____
	_____	_____	_____	_____
	_____	_____	_____	_____
	_____	_____	_____	_____
	_____	_____	_____	_____
	CALORIES :	CALORIES :	CALORIES :	CALORIES :

WEIGHTS & REPS		FATS	CARBS	PROTEINS

FITNESS	WATER IN TAKE	CALORIES	SLEEP TIME	WAKE UP TIME	WEIGHT
MIN / HRS					

MY ACHIEVEMENTS

☐ _____
☐ _____
☐ _____

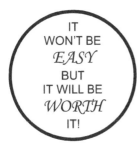

IT
WON'T BE
EASY
BUT
IT WILL BE
WORTH
IT!

WEEKLY CHECK IN

CHECK IN

	M	T	W	T	F	S	S
Drink 8 glasses water	☐	☐	☐	☐	☐	☐	☐
Take my vitamins / supplements	☐	☐	☐	☐	☐	☐	☐
Do my cardio workout	☐	☐	☐	☐	☐	☐	☐
Completed my strength training	☐	☐	☐	☐	☐	☐	☐
Recorded in my food journal	☐	☐	☐	☐	☐	☐	☐
Measured my weight	☐	☐	☐	☐	☐	☐	☐

DID YOU ACCOMPLISH LAST WEEK'S GOALS? IF NOT, WHY?

_____

_____

_____

_____

NEXT WEEK'S GOALS

☐ _____

☐ _____

☐ _____

☐ _____

How I feel today

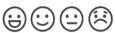

DAY **64**

Date_____

MY COMMITMENTS

_____

_____

_____

FOOD	BREAKFAST	LUNCH	DINNER	SNACKS
	_____	_____	_____	_____
	_____	_____	_____	_____
	_____	_____	_____	_____
	_____	_____	_____	_____
	_____	_____	_____	_____
	CALORIES :	CALORIES :	CALORIES :	CALORIES :

WEIGHTS & REPS		FATS	CARBS	PROTEINS

FITNESS	WATER IN TAKE	CALORIES	SLEEP TIME	WAKE UP TIME	WEIGHT
MIN / HRS					

MY ACHIEVEMENTS

☐ _____

☐ _____

☐ _____

How I feel today

  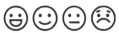

"Strength does not come from the physical capacity. It comes from an indomitable will."
- Gandhi

DAY **65**

Date_____

MY COMMITMENTS

_____
_____
_____

FOOD	BREAKFAST	LUNCH	DINNER	SNACKS
	_____	_____	_____	_____
	_____	_____	_____	_____
	_____	_____	_____	_____
	_____	_____	_____	_____
	_____	_____	_____	_____
	CALORIES :	CALORIES :	CALORIES :	CALORIES :

WEIGHTS & REPS		FATS	CARBS	PROTEINS

FITNESS	WATER IN TAKE	CALORIES	SLEEP TIME	WAKE UP TIME	WEIGHT
MIN / HRS					

MY ACHIEVEMENTS

☐ _____
☐ _____
☐ _____

How I feel today

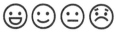

DAY **66**

Date_____

MY COMMITMENTS

_____

_____

_____

FOOD	BREAKFAST	LUNCH	DINNER	SNACKS
	CALORIES :	CALORIES :	CALORIES :	CALORIES :

WEIGHTS & REPS	FATS	CARBS	PROTEINS

FITNESS	WATER IN TAKE	CALORIES	SLEEP TIME	WAKE UP TIME	WEIGHT
MIN / HRS					

MY ACHIEVEMENTS

☐ _____

☐ _____

☐ _____

How I feel today

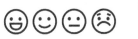

"We are what we repeatedly do.
Excellence then is not an act but a habit."
- Aristotle

DAY **67**

Date_____

MY COMMITMENTS

_____

_____

_____

	BREAKFAST	LUNCH	DINNER	SNACKS
FOOD				
	CALORIES :	CALORIES :	CALORIES :	CALORIES :

WEIGHTS & REPS		FATS	CARBS	PROTEINS

FITNESS	WATER IN TAKE	CALORIES	SLEEP TIME	WAKE UP TIME	WEIGHT
MIN / HRS					

MY ACHIEVEMENTS

☐ _____

☐ _____

☐ _____

How I feel today

"No matter how slow you go,
you are still lapping everybody
on the couch."
- Unknown

DAY **68**

Date_____

MY COMMITMENTS

_____

_____

_____

FOOD	BREAKFAST	LUNCH	DINNER	SNACKS
	_____	_____	_____	_____
	_____	_____	_____	_____
	_____	_____	_____	_____
	_____	_____	_____	_____
	_____	_____	_____	_____
	CALORIES :	CALORIES :	CALORIES :	CALORIES :

WEIGHTS & REPS		FATS	CARBS	PROTEINS

FITNESS	WATER IN TAKE	CALORIES	SLEEP TIME	WAKE UP TIME	WEIGHT
MIN / HRS					

MY ACHIEVEMENTS

☐ _____

☐ _____

☐ _____

How I feel today

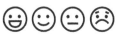

DAY **69**

Date_____

MY COMMITMENTS

_____

_____

_____

	BREAKFAST	LUNCH	DINNER	SNACKS
FOOD	_____	_____	_____	_____
	_____	_____	_____	_____
	_____	_____	_____	_____
	_____	_____	_____	_____
	_____	_____	_____	_____
	CALORIES :	CALORIES :	CALORIES :	CALORIES :

WEIGHTS & REPS		FATS	CARBS	PROTEINS

FITNESS	WATER IN TAKE	CALORIES	SLEEP TIME	WAKE UP TIME	WEIGHT
	🥛🥛🥛🥛🥛🥛🥛				
MIN / HRS					

MY ACHIEVEMENTS

☐ _____

☐ _____

☐ _____

How I feel today

"All great achievements require time."
- Maya Angelon

DAY **70**

Date_____

MY COMMITMENTS

_____
_____
_____

FOOD	BREAKFAST	LUNCH	DINNER	SNACKS
	_____	_____	_____	_____
	_____	_____	_____	_____
	_____	_____	_____	_____
	_____	_____	_____	_____
	_____	_____	_____	_____
	CALORIES :	CALORIES :	CALORIES :	CALORIES :

WEIGHTS & REPS		FATS	CARBS	PROTEINS

FITNESS	WATER IN TAKE	CALORIES	SLEEP TIME	WAKE UP TIME	WEIGHT
	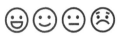				
MIN / HRS					

MY ACHIEVEMENTS

☐ _____
☐ _____
☐ _____

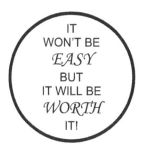

IT WON'T BE *EASY* BUT IT WILL BE *WORTH* IT!

WEEKLY CHECK IN

CHECK IN

	M	T	W	T	F	S	S
Drink 8 glasses water	☐	☐	☐	☐	☐	☐	☐
Take my vitamins / supplements	☐	☐	☐	☐	☐	☐	☐
Do my cardio workout	☐	☐	☐	☐	☐	☐	☐
Completed my strength training	☐	☐	☐	☐	☐	☐	☐
Recorded in my food journal	☐	☐	☐	☐	☐	☐	☐
Measured my weight	☐	☐	☐	☐	☐	☐	☐
	☐	☐	☐	☐	☐	☐	☐

DID YOU ACCOMPLISH LAST WEEK'S GOALS? IF NOT, WHY?

_____

_____

_____

_____

NEXT WEEK'S GOALS

☐ _____

☐ _____

☐ _____

☐ _____

How I feel today

"The difference between try and triumph is a little umph."
- Marvin Phillips

DAY **71**

Date_____

MY COMMITMENTS

_____
_____
_____

FOOD	BREAKFAST	LUNCH	DINNER	SNACKS
	_____	_____	_____	_____
	_____	_____	_____	_____
	_____	_____	_____	_____
	_____	_____	_____	_____
	_____	_____	_____	_____
	CALORIES :	CALORIES :	CALORIES :	CALORIES :

WEIGHTS & REPS		FATS	CARBS	PROTEINS

FITNESS	WATER IN TAKE	CALORIES	SLEEP TIME	WAKE UP TIME	WEIGHT
	🥛🥛🥛🥛🥛🥛🥛				
MIN / HRS					

MY ACHIEVEMENTS

☐ _____
☐ _____
☐ _____

How I feel today

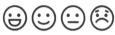

"You only live once, but if you do it right, once is enough."
- Mae West

DAY **72**

Date_____

MY COMMITMENTS

_____

_____

_____

FOOD	BREAKFAST	LUNCH	DINNER	SNACKS
	_____	_____	_____	_____
	_____	_____	_____	_____
	_____	_____	_____	_____
	_____	_____	_____	_____
	_____	_____	_____	_____
	CALORIES :	CALORIES :	CALORIES :	CALORIES :

WEIGHTS & REPS		FATS	CARBS	PROTEINS

FITNESS	WATER IN TAKE	CALORIES	SLEEP TIME	WAKE UP TIME	WEIGHT
MIN / HRS					

MY ACHIEVEMENTS

☐ _____

☐ _____

☐ _____

How I feel today

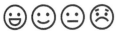

"Passion is energy. Feel the power that comes from focusing on what excites you."
- Oprah Winfrey

DAY **73**

Date_____

MY COMMITMENTS

_____
_____
_____

FOOD	BREAKFAST	LUNCH	DINNER	SNACKS
	_____	_____	_____	_____
	_____	_____	_____	_____
	_____	_____	_____	_____
	_____	_____	_____	_____
	_____	_____	_____	_____
	CALORIES :	CALORIES :	CALORIES :	CALORIES :

WEIGHTS & REPS	FATS	CARBS	PROTEINS

FITNESS	WATER IN TAKE	CALORIES	SLEEP TIME	WAKE UP TIME	WEIGHT
MIN / HRS					

MY ACHIEVEMENTS
- ☐ _____
- ☐ _____
- ☐ _____

How I feel today

😁 🙂 😐 ☹️

DAY **74**

Date_____

MY COMMITMENTS

_____

_____

_____

_____

	BREAKFAST	LUNCH	DINNER	SNACKS
FOOD	_____	_____	_____	_____
	_____	_____	_____	_____
	_____	_____	_____	_____
	_____	_____	_____	_____
	_____	_____	_____	_____
	CALORIES :	CALORIES :	CALORIES :	CALORIES :

WEIGHTS & REPS		FATS	CARBS	PROTEINS

FITNESS	WATER IN TAKE	CALORIES	SLEEP TIME	WAKE UP TIME	WEIGHT
	🥛🥛🥛🥛🥛🥛🥛🥛				
MIN / HRS					

MY ACHIEVEMENTS

☐ _____

☐ _____

☐ _____

How I feel today

  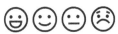

"I believe in pink. I believe that laughing is the best calorie burner."
- Audrey Hepburn

DAY **75**

Date_____

MY COMMITMENTS

_____

_____

_____

FOOD	BREAKFAST	LUNCH	DINNER	SNACKS
	CALORIES :	CALORIES :	CALORIES :	CALORIES :

WEIGHTS & REPS	FATS	CARBS	PROTEINS

FITNESS	WATER IN TAKE	CALORIES	SLEEP TIME	WAKE UP TIME	WEIGHT
MIN / HRS					

MY ACHIEVEMENTS

☐ _____

☐ _____

☐ _____

How I feel today

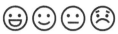

"I believe that tomorrow is another day and I believe in miracles."
- Audrey Hepburn

DAY **76**

Date_____

MY COMMITMENTS

_____
_____
_____

	BREAKFAST	LUNCH	DINNER	SNACKS
FOOD				
	CALORIES :	CALORIES :	CALORIES :	CALORIES :

WEIGHTS & REPS		FATS	CARBS	PROTEINS

FITNESS	WATER IN TAKE	CALORIES	SLEEP TIME	WAKE UP TIME	WEIGHT
MIN / HRS					

MY ACHIEVEMENTS

☐ _____
☐ _____
☐ _____

How I feel today

"When there's that moment of ' Wow, I'm not really sure I can do this,' and you push through those moments, that's when you have a breakthrough."
- Marissa Mayer

DAY **77**

Date_____

MY COMMITMENTS

_____
_____
_____

FOOD	BREAKFAST	LUNCH	DINNER	SNACKS
	CALORIES :	CALORIES :	CALORIES :	CALORIES :

WEIGHTS & REPS		FATS	CARBS	PROTEINS

FITNESS	WATER IN TAKE	CALORIES	SLEEP TIME	WAKE UP TIME	WEIGHT
MIN / HRS					

MY ACHIEVEMENTS

☐ _____
☐ _____
☐ _____

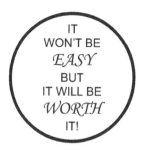

IT
WON'T BE
EASY
BUT
IT WILL BE
WORTH
IT!

WEEKLY CHECK IN

CHECK IN

	M	T	W	T	F	S	S
Drink 8 glasses water	☐	☐	☐	☐	☐	☐	☐
Take my vitamins / supplements	☐	☐	☐	☐	☐	☐	☐
Do my cardio workout	☐	☐	☐	☐	☐	☐	☐
Completed my strength training	☐	☐	☐	☐	☐	☐	☐
Recorded in my food journal	☐	☐	☐	☐	☐	☐	☐
Measured my weight	☐	☐	☐	☐	☐	☐	☐

DID YOU ACCOMPLISH LAST WEEK'S GOALS? IF NOT, WHY?

_____

_____

_____

_____

NEXT WEEK'S GOALS

☐ _____

☐ _____

☐ _____

☐ _____

How I feel today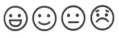

"It is our choices, that show what we truly are, far more than our abilities."
- J.K Rowling

DAY **78**

Date_____

MY COMMITMENTS

_____
_____
_____

FOOD	BREAKFAST	LUNCH	DINNER	SNACKS
	_____	_____	_____	_____
	_____	_____	_____	_____
	_____	_____	_____	_____
	_____	_____	_____	_____
	_____	_____	_____	_____
	CALORIES :	CALORIES :	CALORIES :	CALORIES :

WEIGHTS & REPS		FATS	CARBS	PROTEINS

FITNESS	WATER IN TAKE	CALORIES	SLEEP TIME	WAKE UP TIME	WEIGHT
MIN / HRS					

MY ACHIEVEMENTS

☐ _____
☐ _____
☐ _____

How I feel today

"Our deepest fear is not that we are inadequate. Our deepest fear is that we are powerful beyond measure."
- Marianne Williamson

DAY **79**

Date_____

MY COMMITMENTS

_____
_____
_____

FOOD	BREAKFAST	LUNCH	DINNER	SNACKS
	CALORIES :	CALORIES :	CALORIES :	CALORIES :

WEIGHTS & REPS		FATS	CARBS	PROTEINS

FITNESS	WATER IN TAKE	CALORIES	SLEEP TIME	WAKE UP TIME	WEIGHT
MIN / HRS					

MY ACHIEVEMENTS
☐ _____
☐ _____
☐ _____

How I feel today

"Failure is not the opposite of success, it's part of success."
- Arianna Huffington

DAY **80**

Date_____

MY COMMITMENTS

_____

_____

_____

	BREAKFAST	LUNCH	DINNER	SNACKS
FOOD	_____ _____ _____ _____ _____	_____ _____ _____ _____ _____	_____ _____ _____ _____ _____	_____ _____ _____ _____ _____
	CALORIES :	CALORIES :	CALORIES :	CALORIES :

WEIGHTS & REPS		FATS	CARBS	PROTEINS

FITNESS	WATER IN TAKE	CALORIES	SLEEP TIME	WAKE UP TIME	WEIGHT
MIN / HRS					

MY ACHIEVEMENTS

☐ _____

☐ _____

☐ _____

How I feel today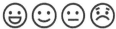

"I'm fearless, I don't complain. Even when horrible things happen to me, I go on."
- Sofia Vergara

DAY **81**

Date_____

MY COMMITMENTS

_____

_____

_____

FOOD	BREAKFAST	LUNCH	DINNER	SNACKS
	_____	_____	_____	_____
	_____	_____	_____	_____
	_____	_____	_____	_____
	_____	_____	_____	_____
	_____	_____	_____	_____
	CALORIES :	CALORIES :	CALORIES :	CALORIES :

WEIGHTS & REPS			FATS	CARBS	PROTEINS

FITNESS	WATER IN TAKE	CALORIES	SLEEP TIME	WAKE UP TIME	WEIGHT
	🥛🥛🥛🥛🥛🥛🥛				
MIN / HRS					

MY ACHIEVEMENTS

☐ _____

☐ _____

☐ _____

How I feel today

"Good things happen to those who hustle."
- Anais Nin

DAY **82**

Date_____

MY COMMITMENTS

_____
_____
_____

	BREAKFAST	LUNCH	DINNER	SNACKS
FOOD	_____ _____ _____ _____ _____	_____ _____ _____ _____ _____	_____ _____ _____ _____ _____	_____ _____ _____ _____ _____
	CALORIES :	CALORIES :	CALORIES :	CALORIES :

WEIGHTS & REPS		FATS	CARBS	PROTEINS

FITNESS	WATER IN TAKE	CALORIES	SLEEP TIME	WAKE UP TIME	WEIGHT
MIN / HRS					

MY ACHIEVEMENTS

- ☐ _____
- ☐ _____
- ☐ _____

How I feel today

"Never let go of that fiery sadness called desire."
- Patti Smith

DAY **83**

Date_____

MY COMMITMENTS

_____

_____

_____

FOOD	BREAKFAST	LUNCH	DINNER	SNACKS
	_____	_____	_____	_____
	_____	_____	_____	_____
	_____	_____	_____	_____
	_____	_____	_____	_____
	_____	_____	_____	_____
	CALORIES :	CALORIES :	CALORIES :	CALORIES :

WEIGHTS & REPS		FATS	CARBS	PROTEINS

FITNESS	WATER IN TAKE	CALORIES	SLEEP TIME	WAKE UP TIME	WEIGHT
	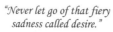				
MIN / HRS					

MY ACHIEVEMENTS
☐ _____
☐ _____
☐ _____

How I feel today

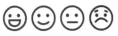

"Challenges are gifts that force us to search for a new center of gravity. Don't fight them. Just find a new way to stand."
- Oprah Winfrey

DAY **84**

Date_____

MY COMMITMENTS

_____
_____
_____
_____

FOOD	BREAKFAST	LUNCH	DINNER	SNACKS
	_____	_____	_____	_____
	_____	_____	_____	_____
	_____	_____	_____	_____
	_____	_____	_____	_____
	_____	_____	_____	_____
	CALORIES :	CALORIES :	CALORIES :	CALORIES :

WEIGHTS & REPS		FATS	CARBS	PROTEINS

FITNESS	WATER IN TAKE	CALORIES	SLEEP TIME	WAKE UP TIME	WEIGHT
MIN / HRS					

MY ACHIEVEMENTS

☐ _____
☐ _____
☐ _____

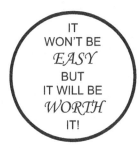

IT
WON'T BE
EASY
BUT
IT WILL BE
WORTH
IT!

WEEKLY CHECK IN

CHECK IN

	M	T	W	T	F	S	S
Drink 8 glasses water	☐	☐	☐	☐	☐	☐	☐
Take my vitamins / supplements	☐	☐	☐	☐	☐	☐	☐
Do my cardio workout	☐	☐	☐	☐	☐	☐	☐
Completed my strength training	☐	☐	☐	☐	☐	☐	☐
Recorded in my food journal	☐	☐	☐	☐	☐	☐	☐
Measured my weight	☐	☐	☐	☐	☐	☐	☐
	☐	☐	☐	☐	☐	☐	☐

DID YOU ACCOMPLISH LAST WEEK'S GOALS? IF NOT, WHY?

_____

_____

_____

_____

NEXT WEEK'S GOALS

☐ _____

☐ _____

☐ _____

☐ _____

How I feel today

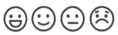

DAY **85**

Date_____

MY COMMITMENTS

_____

_____

_____

	BREAKFAST	LUNCH	DINNER	SNACKS
FOOD	_____	_____	_____	_____
	_____	_____	_____	_____
	_____	_____	_____	_____
	_____	_____	_____	_____
	_____	_____	_____	_____
	CALORIES :	CALORIES :	CALORIES :	CALORIES :

WEIGHTS & REPS		FATS	CARBS	PROTEINS

FITNESS	WATER IN TAKE	CALORIES	SLEEP TIME	WAKE UP TIME	WEIGHT
	🥛🥛🥛🥛🥛🥛🥛				
MIN / HRS					

MY ACHIEVEMENTS

☐ _____

☐ _____

☐ _____

How I feel today

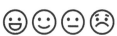

*"You gotta run more than your mouth
to escape the treadmill of mediocrity."*
- **Jarod Kintz**

DAY **86**

Date_____

MY COMMITMENTS

_____
_____
_____

FOOD	BREAKFAST	LUNCH	DINNER	SNACKS
	_____	_____	_____	_____
	_____	_____	_____	_____
	_____	_____	_____	_____
	_____	_____	_____	_____
	_____	_____	_____	_____
	CALORIES :	CALORIES :	CALORIES :	CALORIES :

WEIGHTS & REPS		FATS	CARBS	PROTEINS

FITNESS	WATER IN TAKE	CALORIES	SLEEP TIME	WAKE UP TIME	WEIGHT
MIN / HRS	🥛🥛🥛🥛🥛🥛🥛🥛				

MY ACHIEVEMENTS

☐ _____
☐ _____
☐ _____

How I feel today

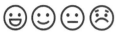

"I've got a dream that's worth more than my sleep."
- Unknown

_____ DAY **87**

Date_____

MY COMMITMENTS

_____
_____
_____

FOOD	BREAKFAST	LUNCH	DINNER	SNACKS
	CALORIES :	CALORIES :	CALORIES :	CALORIES :

WEIGHTS & REPS		FATS	CARBS	PROTEINS

FITNESS	WATER IN TAKE	CALORIES	SLEEP TIME	WAKE UP TIME	WEIGHT
MIN / HRS					

MY ACHIEVEMENTS

- [ ] _____
- [ ] _____
- [ ] _____

How I feel today

"The struggle you're in today is developing the strength you need for tomorrow. Don't give up."
- **Robert Tew**

DAY **88**

Date_____

MY COMMITMENTS

_____

_____

_____

FOOD	BREAKFAST	LUNCH	DINNER	SNACKS
	_____	_____	_____	_____
	_____	_____	_____	_____
	_____	_____	_____	_____
	_____	_____	_____	_____
	_____	_____	_____	_____
	CALORIES :	CALORIES :	CALORIES :	CALORIES :

WEIGHTS & REPS		FATS	CARBS	PROTEINS

FITNESS	WATER IN TAKE	CALORIES	SLEEP TIME	WAKE UP TIME	WEIGHT
MIN / HRS					

MY ACHIEVEMENTS

☐ _____

☐ _____

☐ _____

How I feel today

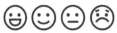

"It takes as much energy to wish as it does to plan."
- Eleanor Roosevelt

DAY **89**

Date_____

MY COMMITMENTS

_____

_____

_____

FOOD	BREAKFAST	LUNCH	DINNER	SNACKS
	_____	_____	_____	_____
	_____	_____	_____	_____
	_____	_____	_____	_____
	_____	_____	_____	_____
	_____	_____	_____	_____
	CALORIES :	CALORIES :	CALORIES :	CALORIES :

WEIGHTS & REPS		FATS	CARBS	PROTEINS

FITNESS	WATER IN TAKE	CALORIES	SLEEP TIME	WAKE UP TIME	WEIGHT
MIN / HRS					

MY ACHIEVEMENTS

☐ _____

☐ _____

☐ _____

How I feel today

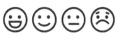

"If you're going through hell, keep going."
- Winston Churchill

DAY **90**

Date_____

MY COMMITMENTS

_____
_____
_____
_____

	BREAKFAST	LUNCH	DINNER	SNACKS
FOOD	_____	_____	_____	_____
	_____	_____	_____	_____
	_____	_____	_____	_____
	_____	_____	_____	_____
	_____	_____	_____	_____
	CALORIES :	CALORIES :	CALORIES :	CALORIES :

WEIGHTS & REPS		FATS	CARBS	PROTEINS

FITNESS	WATER IN TAKE	CALORIES	SLEEP TIME	WAKE UP TIME	WEIGHT
	🥛🥛🥛🥛🥛🥛🥛				
MIN / HRS					

MY ACHIEVEMENTS

☐ _____
☐ _____
☐ _____

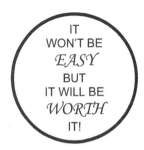

IT WON'T BE *EASY* BUT IT WILL BE *WORTH* IT!

WEEKLY CHECK IN

CHECK IN							
	M	T	W	T	F	S	S
Drink 8 glasses water	☐	☐	☐	☐	☐	☐	☐
Take my vitamins / supplements	☐	☐	☐	☐	☐	☐	☐
Do my cardio workout	☐	☐	☐	☐	☐	☐	☐
Completed my strength training	☐	☐	☐	☐	☐	☐	☐
Recorded in my food journal	☐	☐	☐	☐	☐	☐	☐
Measured my weight	☐	☐	☐	☐	☐	☐	☐

DID YOU ACCOMPLISH LAST WEEK'S GOALS? IF NOT, WHY?

_____

_____

_____

_____

NEXT WEEK'S GOALS

☐ _____

☐ _____

☐ _____

☐ _____

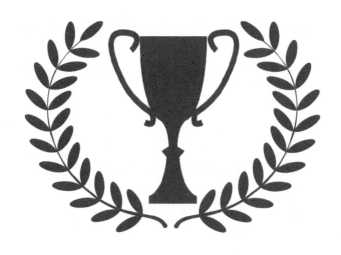

Congratulations

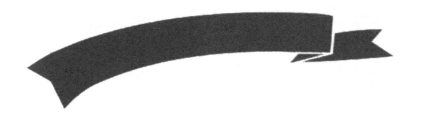

★★★★★

YOU DID IT!

SIGN UP TO GET YOUR COMPLETION CERTIFICATE

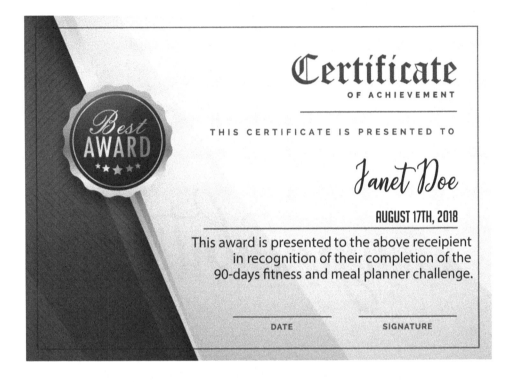

VISIT THE BELOW ADDRESS TO RECEIVE YOUR PERSONALIZED
CERTIFICATE OF COMPLETION

https://www.facebook.com/groups/rimsportsvip/

Made in USA - Kendallville, IN
91623_9781718144828
02.09.2022 1516